EASY DIABETIC SMOOTHIE RECIPES

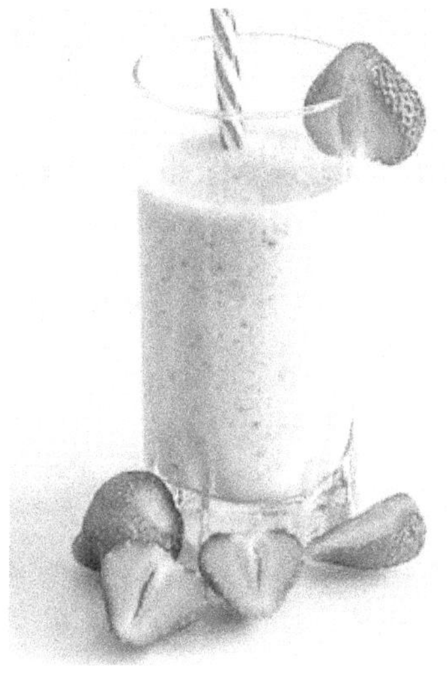

31 Quick and Simple Low Sugar Smoothie Recipes for Diabetes

EVELYN T. LATTORE

The recipes and the information contained in this cookbook are intended to provide helpful and informative material on the subjects addressed. The information contained herein is not intended to substitute for advice given by a medical professional. Before starting any diet or exercise program, seek medical advice.

If you have any question, I'll be available to help; you can reach me via dietwithevelyn@gmail.com

Other Books by Publisher:

Diabetes Dessert Cookbook

The Complete Diabetic Cookbook for Seniors

Type 1 Diabetes Cookbook for Kids

Diabetic Air fryer Cookbook

Diabetic Cookbook for Beginners

TABLE OF CONTENT

Pomegranate Smoothie

Chocolate Hazelnut Smoothie

Mango Coconut Smoothie

Chia Berry Smoothie

Green Lemonade Smoothie

Apple Pie Smoothie

Peach Yogurt Smoothie

Coconut Mango Smoothie

Banana Kale Smoothie

Orange Avocado Smoothie

Blueberry Almond Smoothie

Cacao Banana Smoothie

Pineapple Coconut Smoothie

Almond Butter Smoothie

Speak To Your Body

INTRODUCTION

Controlling your blood sugar levels is crucial for your health if you have diabetes. One way to do this is to eat a healthy diet that is low in carbohydrates and high in fiber. Smoothies can be a great way to fit more fruits, vegetables, and whole grains into your diet, while also keeping your blood sugar levels in check.

This book is a collection of 31 diabetic-friendly smoothie recipes that are both delicious and nutritious. Each recipe includes a list of ingredients, and step-by-step instructions. Whether you are looking for a quick and easy breakfast or a refreshing snack, you will find a recipe in this book that you will love.

In addition to being delicious, smoothies are also a great way to get your daily dose of fruits and vegetables. Fruits and vegetables provide a variety of vitamins, minerals, and antioxidants that are essential for good health. They can also help to lower your blood sugar levels and reduce your risk of developing other chronic diseases.

Smoothies are also a great way to lose weight or maintain a healthy weight. They are low in calories and fat, and they can help you to feel full longer. If you are trying to lose weight, aim to drink one or two smoothies per day.

If you have diabetes, smoothies can be a great addition to your diet. They are a delicious, nutritious, and convenient way to get the nutrients you need to stay healthy.

Here are some tips for making smoothies for diabetes:

Use low-glycemic index fruits and vegetables. These fruits and vegetables have a slower impact on blood sugar levels. Some good choices include berries, apples, pears, carrots, and spinach.

Avoid sweetening your smoothies with sugar. Instead, use natural sweeteners like stevia or monk fruit extract.

Add protein powder to your smoothies. Protein can help to keep you feeling full longer and can also help to stabilize blood sugar levels.

Add healthy fats to your smoothies. Healthy fats like avocado, nuts, and seeds can help to slow down the absorption of sugar into the bloodstream.

Experiment with different flavors and ingredients. The possibilities for making smoothies are essentially endless. So get creative and have fun!

Benefits of drinking smoothies as a diabetic:

There are many benefits to drinking smoothies as a diabetic. Smoothies can help to:

Improve blood sugar control. Fruits and vegetables are low on the glycemic index, which means that they release sugar into the bloodstream slowly. This may lessen the likelihood of post-meal blood sugar increases.

Increase fiber intake. Fiber helps slow down sugar absorption into the bloodstream, which can also help prevent blood sugar spikes.

Boost weight loss. Smoothies can be a great way to add more fruits, vegetables, and whole grains to your diet, which can help you to lose weight or maintain a healthy weight.

Provide essential nutrients. The vitamins, and antioxidants found in fruits and vegetables are vital for maintaining excellent health.

Make mealtimes easier. Smoothies can be a quick and easy way to get a healthy meal or snack. You may carry them with you everywhere you go because they are also portable.

If you have diabetes, smoothies can be a great addition to your diet. Just be sure to choose recipes that are low in sugar and high in fiber. You may also want to add a source of protein, such as yogurt or protein powder, to your smoothies.

Let's get started!

Berry Blast Smoothie

Ingredients

-1/2 cup fresh blueberries

-1/2 cup fresh raspberries

-1/2 cup fresh blackberries

-1/2 cup low-fat Greek yogurt

-1/4 cup orange juice

-1 tablespoon honey

-1/2 teaspoon cinnamon

-1/2 cup crushed ice

Method

1. In a blender, combine blueberries, raspberries, blackberries, yogurt, orange juice, honey, and cinnamon.

2. Blend until smooth.

3. To achieve the correct consistency, add crushed ice and blend once more.

4. Pour into a glass and enjoy!

Mango Pineapple Smoothie

Ingredients

-1/2 cup diced mango

-1/2 cup diced pineapple

-1/2 cup low-fat Greek yogurt

-1 tablespoon honey

-1/2 teaspoon turmeric

-1/2 cup crushed ice

Method

1. In a blender, combine mango, pineapple, yogurt, honey, and turmeric.

2. Blend until smooth.

3. To achieve the correct consistency, add crushed ice and blend once more.

4. Pour into a glass and enjoy!

Tropical Green Smoothie

Ingredients

-1/2 cup diced mango

-1/2 cup diced pineapple

-1/2 cup baby spinach

-1/2 cup low-fat Greek yogurt

-1/4 cup orange juice

-1 tablespoon honey

-1/2 cup crushed ice

Method

1. In a blender, combine mango, pineapple, spinach, yogurt, orange juice, and honey.

2. Blend until smooth.

3. To achieve the correct consistency, add crushed ice and blend once more.

4. Pour into a glass and enjoy!

Peachy Almond Smoothie

Ingredients

-1/2 cup diced peaches

-1/4 cup almond milk

-1/4 cup low-fat Greek yogurt

-1 tablespoon honey

-1/2 teaspoon ground ginger

-1/2 cup crushed ice

Method

1. In a blender, combine peaches, almond milk, yogurt, honey, and ginger.

2. Blend until smooth.

3. To achieve the correct consistency, add crushed ice and blend once more.

4. Pour into a glass and enjoy!

Chocolate Banana Smoothie

Ingredients

-1/2 cup diced banana

-1/4 cup almond milk

-1/4 cup low-fat Greek yogurt

-1 tablespoon cocoa powder

-1 tablespoon honey

-1/2 cup crushed ice

Method

1. In a blender, combine banana, almond milk, yogurt, cocoa powder, and honey.

2. Blend until smooth.

3. To achieve the correct consistency, add crushed ice and blend once more.

4. Pour into a glass and enjoy!

Orange Dream Smoothie

Ingredients

-1/2 cup diced oranges

-1/4 cup almond milk

-1/4 cup low-fat Greek yogurt

-1 tablespoon honey

-1/2 teaspoon ground cinnamon

-1/2 cup crushed ice

Method

1. In a blender, combine oranges, almond milk, yogurt, honey, and cinnamon.

2. Blend until smooth.

3. To achieve the correct consistency, add crushed ice and blend once more.

4. Pour into a glass and enjoy!

Carrot Cake Smoothie

Ingredients

-1/2 cup diced carrots

-1/4 cup almond milk

-1/4 cup low-fat Greek yogurt

-1 tablespoon honey

-1/2 teaspoon ground nutmeg

-1/2 cup crushed ice

Method

1. In a blender, combine carrots, almond milk, yogurt, honey, and nutmeg.

2. Blend until smooth.

3. To achieve the correct consistency, add crushed ice and blend once more.

4. Pour into a glass and enjoy!

Apple Spice Smoothie

Ingredients

-1/2 cup diced apples

-1/4 cup almond milk

-1/4 cup low-fat Greek yogurt

-1 tablespoon honey

-1/2 teaspoon ground cinnamon

-1/2 cup crushed ice

Method

1. In a blender, combine apples, almond milk, yogurt, honey, and cinnamon.

2. Blend until smooth.

3. To achieve the correct consistency, add crushed ice and blend once more.

4. Pour into a glass and enjoy!

Beet Berry Smoothie

Ingredients

-1/2 cup diced beets

-1/2 cup frozen berries

-1/2 cup low-fat Greek yogurt

-1 tablespoon honey

-1/2 teaspoon ground cinnamon

-1/2 cup crushed ice

Method

1. In a blender, combine beets, berries, yogurt, honey, and cinnamon.

2. Blend until smooth.

3. To achieve the correct consistency, add crushed ice and blend once more.

4. Pour into a glass and enjoy!

Banana Oat Smoothie

Ingredients

-1/2 cup diced banana

-1/4 cup rolled oats

-1/4 cup almond milk

-1 tablespoon honey

-1/2 teaspoon ground cinnamon

-1/2 cup crushed ice

Method

1. In a blender, combine banana, oats, almond milk, honey, and cinnamon.

2. Blend until smooth.

3. To achieve the correct consistency, add crushed ice and blend once more.

4. Pour into a glass and enjoy!

Green Tea Smoothie

Ingredients

-1/2 cup diced mango

-1/4 cup green tea

-1/4 cup low-fat Greek yogurt

-1 tablespoon honey

-1/2 teaspoon matcha powder

-1/2 cup crushed ice

Method

1. In a blender, combine mango, green tea, yogurt, honey, and matcha powder.

2. Blend until smooth.

3. To achieve the correct consistency, add crushed ice and blend once more.

4. Pour into a glass and enjoy!

Avocado Smoothie

Ingredients

-1/2 cup diced avocado

-1/4 cup almond milk

-1/4 cup low-fat Greek yogurt

-1 tablespoon honey

-1/2 teaspoon ground cardamom

-1/2 cup crushed ice

Method

1. In a blender, combine avocado, almond milk, yogurt, honey, and cardamom.

2. Blend until smooth.

3. To achieve the correct consistency, add crushed ice and blend once more.

4. Pour into a glass and enjoy!

Cucumber Mint Smoothie

Ingredients

-1/2 cup diced cucumber

-1/4 cup almond milk

-1/4 cup low-fat Greek yogurt

-1 tablespoon honey

-1/2 teaspoon mint extract

-1/2 cup crushed ice

Method

1. In a blender, combine cucumber, almond milk, yogurt, honey, and mint extract.

2. Blend until smooth.

3. To achieve the correct consistency, add crushed ice and blend once more.

4. Pour into a glass and enjoy!

Caramel Apple Smoothie

Ingredients

-1/2 cup diced apples

-1/4 cup almond milk

-1/4 cup low-fat Greek yogurt

-1 tablespoon caramel syrup

-1/2 teaspoon ground cinnamon

-1/2 cup crushed ice

Method

1. In a blender, combine apples, almond milk, yogurt, caramel syrup, and cinnamon.

2. Blend until smooth.

3. To achieve the correct consistency, add crushed ice and blend once more.

4. Pour into a glass and enjoy!

Mixed Berry Smoothie

Ingredients

-1/2 cup frozen mixed berries

-1/4 cup almond milk

-1/4 cup low-fat Greek yogurt

-1 tablespoon honey

-1/2 teaspoon ground ginger

-1/2 cup crushed ice

Method

1. In a blender, combine mixed berries, almond milk, yogurt, honey, and ginger.

2. Blend until smooth.

3. To achieve the correct consistency, add crushed ice and blend once more.

4. Pour into a glass and enjoy!

Kiwi Coconut Smoothie

Ingredients

-1/2 cup diced kiwi

-1/4 cup coconut milk

-1/4 cup low-fat Greek yogurt

-1 tablespoon honey

-1/2 teaspoon ground cardamom

-1/2 cup crushed ice

Method

Method

1. In a blender, combine kiwi, coconut milk, yogurt, honey, and cardamom.

2. Blend until smooth.

3. To achieve the correct consistency, add crushed ice and blend once more.

4. Pour into a glass and enjoy!

Banana Almond Smoothie

Ingredients

-1/2 cup diced banana

-1/4 cup almond milk

-1/4 cup low-fat Greek yogurt

-1 tablespoon almond butter

-1/2 teaspoon ground cinnamon

-1/2 cup crushed ice

Method

1. In a blender, combine banana, almond milk, yogurt, almond butter, and cinnamon.

2. Blend until smooth.

3. To achieve the correct consistency, add crushed ice and blend once more.

4. Pour into a glass and enjoy!

Pomegranate Smoothie

Ingredients

-1/2 cup pomegranate seeds

-1/4 cup almond milk

-1/4 cup low-fat Greek yogurt

-1 tablespoon honey

-1/2 teaspoon ground cardamom

-1/2 cup crushed ice

Method

1. In a blender, combine pomegranate seeds, almond milk, yogurt, honey, and cardamom.

2. Blend until smooth.

3. To achieve the correct consistency, add crushed ice and blend once more.

4. Pour into a glass and enjoy!

Chocolate Hazelnut Smoothie

Ingredients

-1/4 cup almond milk

-1/4 cup low-fat Greek yogurt

-1 tablespoon cocoa powder

-1 tablespoon hazelnut butter

-1 tablespoon honey

-1/2 cup crushed ice

Method

1. In a blender, combine almond milk, yogurt, cocoa powder, hazelnut butter, and honey.

2. Blend until smooth.

3. To achieve the correct consistency, add crushed ice and blend once more..

4. Pour into a glass and enjoy!

Mango Coconut Smoothie

Ingredients

-1/2 cup diced mango

-1/4 cup coconut milk

-1/4 cup low-fat Greek yogurt

-1 tablespoon honey

-1/2 teaspoon ground turmeric

-1/2 cup crushed ice

Method

1. In a blender, combine mango, coconut milk, yogurt, honey, and turmeric.

2. Blend until smooth.

3. To achieve the correct consistency, add crushed ice and blend once more.

4. Pour into a glass and enjoy!

Chia Berry Smoothie

Ingredients

-1/2 cup frozen mixed berries

-1/4 cup almond milk

-1/4 cup low-fat Greek yogurt

-1 tablespoon honey

-1 tablespoon chia seeds

-1/2 cup crushed ice

Method

1. In a blender, combine mixed berries, almond milk, yogurt, honey, and chia seeds.

2. Blend until smooth.

3. To achieve the correct consistency, add crushed ice and blend once more.

4. Pour into a glass and enjoy!

Green Lemonade Smoothie

Ingredients

-1/2 cup baby spinach

-1/4 cup almond milk

-1/4 cup low-fat Greek yogurt

-1 tablespoon honey

-1/2 teaspoon ground ginger

-1/2 cup crushed ice

Method

1. In a blender, combine spinach, almond milk, yogurt, honey, and ginger.

2. Blend until smooth.

3. To achieve the correct consistency, add crushed ice and blend once more.

4. Pour into a glass and enjoy!

Apple Pie Smoothie

Ingredients

-1/2 cup diced apples

-1/4 cup almond milk

-1/4 cup low-fat Greek yogurt

-1 tablespoon honey

-1/2 teaspoon ground nutmeg

-1/2 cup crushed ice

Method

1. In a blender, combine apples, almond milk, yogurt, honey, and nutmeg.

2. Blend until smooth.

3. To achieve the correct consistency, add crushed ice and blend once more.

4. Pour into a glass and enjoy!

Peach Yogurt Smoothie

Ingredients

-1/2 cup diced peaches

-1/4 cup almond milk

-1/4 cup low-fat Greek yogurt

-1 tablespoon honey

-1/2 teaspoon ground cardamom

-1/2 cup crushed ice

Method

1. In a blender, combine peaches, almond milk, yogurt, honey, and cardamom.

2. Blend until smooth.

3. To achieve the correct consistency, add crushed ice and blend once more.

4. Pour into a glass and enjoy!

Coconut Mango Smoothie

Ingredients

-1/2 cup diced mango

-1/4 cup coconut milk

-1/4 cup low-fat Greek yogurt

-1 tablespoon honey

-1/2 teaspoon ground ginger

-1/2 cup crushed ice

Method

1. In a blender, combine mango, coconut milk, yogurt, honey, and ginger.

2. Blend until smooth.

3. To achieve the correct consistency, add crushed ice and blend once more.

4. Pour into a glass and enjoy!

Banana Kale Smoothie

Ingredients

-1/2 cup diced banana

-1/2 cup baby kale

-1/2 cup low-fat Greek yogurt

-1 tablespoon honey

-1/2 teaspoon ground cinnamon

-1/2 cup crushed ice

Method

1. In a blender, combine banana, kale, yogurt, honey, and cinnamon.

2. Blend until smooth.

3. To achieve the correct consistency, add crushed ice and blend once more.

4. Pour into a glass and enjoy!

Orange Avocado Smoothie

Ingredients

-1/2 cup diced oranges

-1/2 cup diced avocado

-1/2 cup low-fat Greek yogurt

-1 tablespoon honey

-1/2 teaspoon ground nutmeg

-1/2 cup crushed ice

Method

1. In a blender, combine oranges, avocado, yogurt, honey, and nutmeg.

2. Blend until smooth.

3. To achieve the correct consistency, add crushed ice and blend once more.

4. Pour into a glass and enjoy!

Blueberry Almond Smoothie

Ingredients

-1/2 cup fresh blueberries

-1/4 cup almond milk

-1/4 cup low-fat Greek yogurt

-1 tablespoon honey

-1/2 teaspoon ground cardamom

-1/2 cup crushed ice

Method

1. In a blender, combine blueberries, almond milk, yogurt, honey, and cardamom.

2. Blend until smooth.

3. To achieve the correct consistency, add crushed ice and blend once more.

4. Pour into a glass and enjoy!

Cacao Banana Smoothie

Ingredients

-1/2 cup diced banana

-1/4 cup almond milk

-1/4 cup low-fat Greek yogurt

-1 tablespoon cacao powder

-1 tablespoon honey

-1/2 cup crushed ice

Method

1. In a blender, combine banana, almond milk, yogurt, cacao powder, and honey.

2. Blend until smooth.

3. To achieve the correct consistency, add crushed ice and blend once more.

4. Pour into a glass and enjoy!

Pineapple Coconut Smoothie

Ingredients

-1/2 cup diced pineapple

-1/4 cup coconut milk

-1/4 cup low-fat Greek yogurt

-1 tablespoon honey

-1/2 teaspoon ground ginger

-1/2 cup crushed ice

Method

1. In a blender, combine pineapple, coconut milk, yogurt, honey, and ginger.

2. Blend until smooth.

3. To achieve the correct consistency, add crushed ice and blend once more.

4. Pour into a glass and enjoy!

Almond Butter Smoothie

Ingredients

-1/2 cup diced banana

-1/4 cup almond milk

-1/4 cup low-fat Greek yogurt

-1 tablespoon almond butter

-1 tablespoon honey

-1/2 cup crushed ice

Method

1. In a blender, combine banana, almond milk, yogurt, almond butter, and honey.

2. Blend until smooth.

3. To achieve the correct consistency, add crushed ice and blend once more.

4. Pour into a glass and enjoy!

I am made whole through the love and grace of Jesus.

I am living my best life even with diabetes.

I will take control of my health and make healthy choices that are tailored to my specific needs.

My glucose levels are stable and I am feeling vibrant and strong.

I am confident in my ability to make positive changes in my life that will help me manage my diabetes.

I honor my body and recognize the importance of self-care.

I respect and love myself and I know that I am capable of living a life of good health and wellness, despite the challenges of diabetes.

I believe in Jesus and in the power of His resurrection to bring healing and strength to my body.

I accept Him as my Lord and saviour and I trust that He will guide me on my journey to wellness. Amen.